ISBN-13: 978-0615833750
Author: Robert Johnson

This publication is designed to provide accurate and authoritative information in regard to the subject matter covered. It is sold with the understanding that the publisher is not engaged in rendering legal, accounting or other professional services. If legal advice or other professional assistance is required, the services of a competent professional person should be sought.

- From a Declaration of Principles jointly adopted by a Committee of the American Bar Association and a Committee of Publishers and Associations.

No responsibility or liability is assumed by the Publisher for any injury, damage or financial loss sustained to persons or property from the use of this information, personal or otherwise, either directly or indirectly. While every effort has been made to ensure reliability and accuracy of the information within, all liability, negligence or otherwise, from any use, misuse or abuse of the operation of any methods, strategies, instructions or ideas contained in the material herein, is the sole responsibility of the reader.

All information is generalized, presented for informational purposes only and presented "as is" without warranty or guarantee of any kind.

All trademarks and brands referred to in this book are for illustrative purposes only, are the property of their respective owners and not affiliated with this publication in any way. Any trademarks are being used without permission, and the publication of the trademark is not authorized by, associated with or sponsored by the trademark owner.

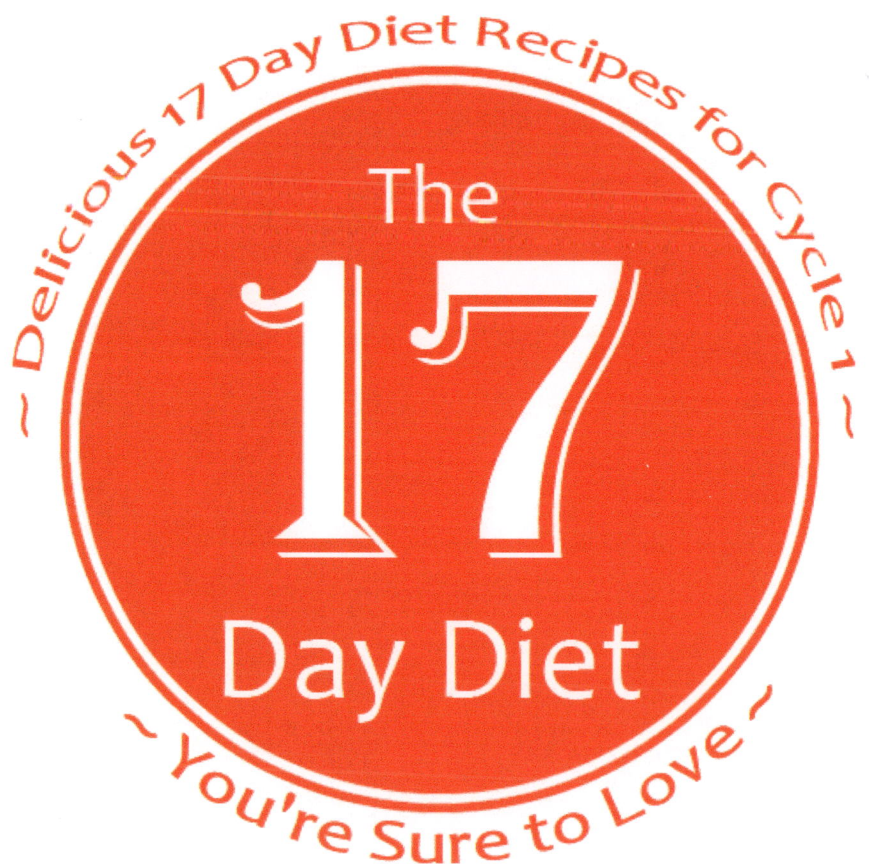
~ Delicious 17 Day Diet Recipes for Cycle 1 ~
The
17
Day Diet
~ You're Sure to Love ~

Summary

This report consists primarily of two portions. The first of which involves a short introduction and description of the *17 Day Diet*, a dietary plan proposed by family physician, Dr. Mike Moreno. It was first made popular when it was featured on the TV show Doctors, hosted by none other than the esteemed, Dr. Phil.

The 17 Day Diet involves four cycles. However, this report will mainly focus on providing recipes applicable for the first cycle. There are a total of 30 recipes presented. All of which adhere to the 17 day diet's strict regulations. We sincerely hope that these recipes help make a significant impact on your health and overall quality of life. Enjoy yourself and good luck with your diet!

Table of Contents

Introduction

What is the 17 day diet?

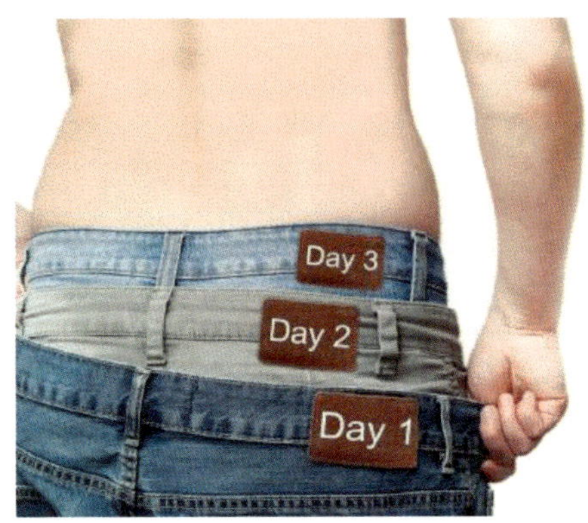

The 17 Day Diet is the brainchild of Dr. Mike Moreno, a family physician based in California. The dietary plan owes much of its popularity to being featured on the popular TV show, The Doctors, hosted by none other than Dr. Phil. In fact, it is so popular that it can be considered one of the hottest trending dietary plans practiced today.

Dr. Moreno's diet operates on the premise that the weight gain is not only caused by overeating and a series of poor food choices, but also by the body's propensity to adapt to the regular intake of the same types of food. The dietary plan aims to break this cycle of, so called, "metabolic confusion" by proposing a 17 day meal schedule consisting of very different varieties of food.

Although the diet was originally intended to be followed during the holidays, when people tend to gain a few extra pounds, Dr. Moreno states that it can actually be used during any period of the year. It has been widely hailed as an effective method to rapidly reduce body fat and excess weight. In fact, some may suggest that it is possible to lose 10 to 12 pounds within the first few days.

To fully enjoy the benefits of Dr. Moreno's dietary plan, you should complete all of its 4 cycles. Each cycle lasts for a total of 17 days. These relatively short cycles mean that practitioners of the diet have easy-to-achieve benchmarks where they can draw positive reinforcement from. This, in turn, motivates them to continue with the dietary plan.

The 4 cycles

Although this report will mainly cover only the 1st cycle of the Dr. Moreno's diet, it is still important to understand all you can about the full dietary plan. This will not only help you better appreciate the 17 Day Diet, but will also help you make an informed decision as to whether or not you will ultimately finish the entire plan. Here is a short summary of each 17-day cycle.

Cycle 1: Accelerate. The 1st phase of the diet involves drastically reducing the amount of calories you ingest per day. By reducing your calorie intake, especially those gained from carbohydrate-rich food, you promote fat burning, bodily cleansing, and weight loss.

Cycle 2: Activate. This phase aims to modify the old metabolism of your body by calorie shifting. This means that you a varied amount of calories every day. The purpose of doing such is to keep your body's metabolism on its toes and prevent it from slowing down.

Cycle 3: Achieve. Here you will start reintroducing previously restricted foods into your diet. The aim of this stage is to develop the healthy eating habits that you can practice even after the full completion of the dietary plan

Cycle 4: Arrive. This final phase in the plan allows you to splurge a bit during weekends. During such time you can indulge in all your favorite foods, but on the promise that you will return to your healthy eating habits on the weekdays.

17 Day Diet Recipes – Cycle 1

The following recipes discussed can all be used for the 1st phase of the 17 Day Diet. The foods made from these recipes are all low-carb and mostly fat-free. While eating these foods, you should ideally consume only 1200 calories a day.

Awesome Apple Chips

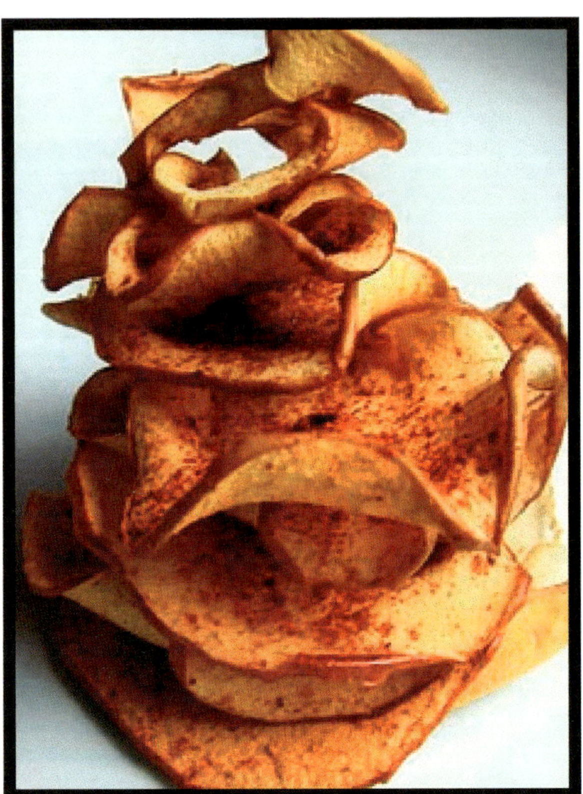

Ingredients:

- 2 apples
- ½ tsp. cinnamon
- 2 packets artificial sweetener
- Non-stick cooking spray

Procedure:

1. Preheat oven to 300°F.
2. Coat a cookie sheet with the cooking spray.
3. Peel and core the apples.

4. Slice the apples. The thinner the better. Ideally, you will want to use a paring knife or mandolin.
5. Mix the cinnamon and artificial sweetener in a small bowl.
6. Place the apples on the baking sheet.
7. Sprinkle the slices with the contents of the small bowl.
8. Bake until crispy. The process takes around 45 minutes.
9. Remove from the oven and let cool.
10. Indulge!

Broccoli Chicken Dijon

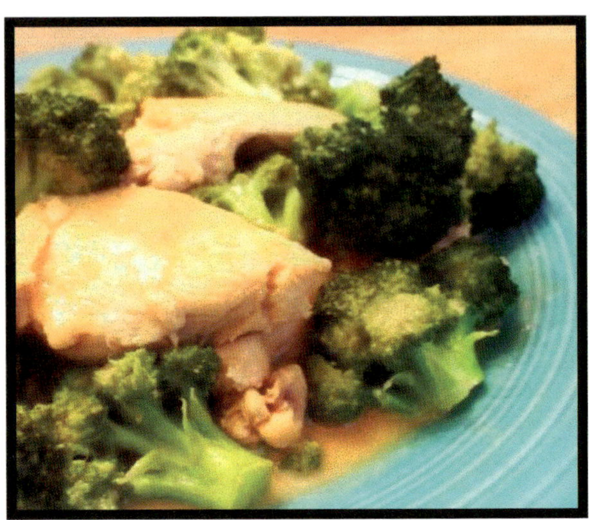

Ingredients:

½ cup chicken broth
1 tbsp. soy sauce
4 cups broccoli, shredded into florets
1 clove garlic, minced
1 tbsp. olive oil
1 lb. boneless chicken breast, skinned, thinly sliced
2 tbsp. Dijon mustard

Procedure:

1. In a large bowl, mix the chicken broth and soy sauce.
2. Pour the olive oil into a large skillet and heat over medium-high heat.
3. Cook the broccoli and garlic in the skillet. Remember to stir continuously.
4. Remove them from the skillet and set aside.
5. Cook the chicken in the skillet for around 4 minutes or until cooked thoroughly.
6. Pour in the chicken broth mixture.

7. Increase the heat and bring to the ingredients the broth to a boil.
8. Reduce the heat to medium-low.
9. Pour in the mustard and mix until thoroughly combined
10. Add the cooked broccoli and garlic. Continue stirring.
11. Cook for a few more minutes or until heated through. Remember to stir occasionally.
12. Plate and serve.

Cajun Baked Fish

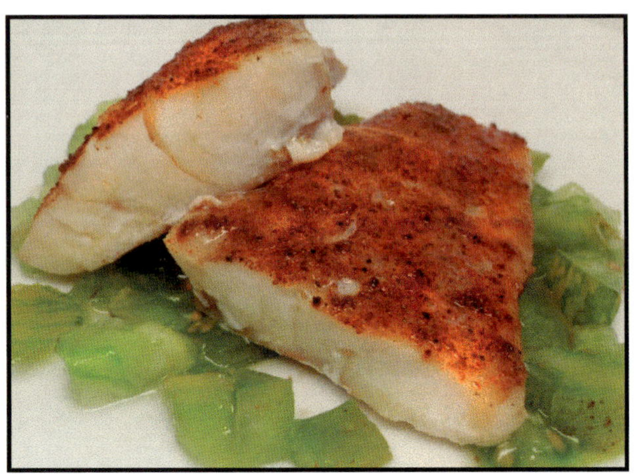

Ingredients:

- 1 tbsp. olive oil
- ½ tsp. garlic powder
- ½ tsp. sea salt
- 2 tsp. thyme, dried
- 2 tsp. paprika
- ¼ tsp. cayenne peppers, crushed
- ½ tsp. hot sauce
- ¼ tsp. black pepper
- 4 8oz. fillets of catfish, optional alternatives: tilapia or tuna
- Non-stick cooking spray
- Aluminum foil

Preparation:

1. Preheat the oven to 425°F.
2. Set aside the fish, black pepper, cooking spray, and aluminum foil.
3. Combine all the other ingredients in a small bowl.
4. Brush the contents of the small bowl on the sides of each fillet.
5. Cut the aluminum foil into pieces big enough to completely cover each fillet.
6. Coat the aluminum foil pieces with the cooking spray.

7. Wrap each coated fillet with an aluminum foil piece.
8. Place the wrapped fillets on a baking pan.
9. Bake for 13 minutes or until fish flakes easily.

Caribbean Chicken

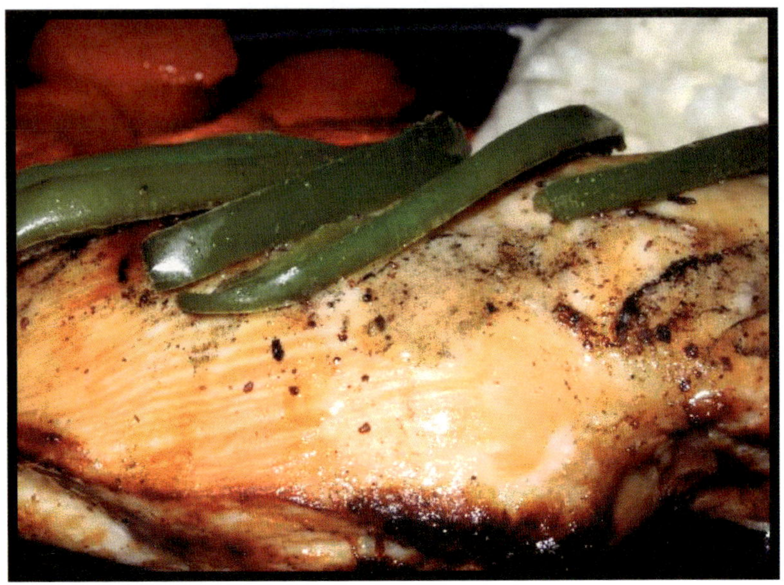

Ingredients:

4 boneless chicken breasts, skinned
3 jalapeno peppers, sliced
3 cloves garlic, minced
½ cup vinegar
½ cup soy sauce
½ tsp. cinnamon
½ tsp. nutmeg
1 pinch ground cloves
1 pinch sea salt
1 pinch black pepper

Procedure:

1. Set aside the chicken breasts
2. In a large bowl, mix all the other ingredients.
3. Coat the chicken breasts with the mixture.
4. Marinate overnight.

5. Cook the chicken in whatever way you like. Kabobs on the grill are recommended.
6. Be creative and enjoy!

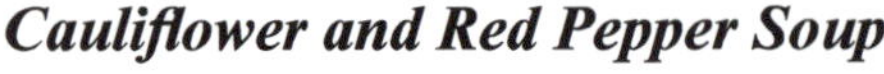

Cauliflower and Red Pepper Soup

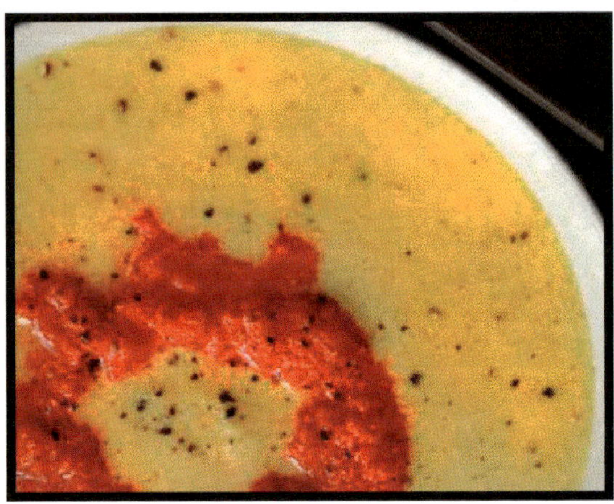

Ingredients:

Cauliflower soup

- 1 head cauliflower, shredded into florets
- 2 tbsp. olive oil
- 1 onion, chopped
- 4 cups chicken broth
- 2 cloves garlic, minced
- 1 tsp. orange juice
- Sea salt and black pepper to taste

Red pepper puree

- ½ cup roasted red peppers
- 1 tbsp. olive oil
- 1 tsp. lemon juice

Procedure:

1. Place the peppers, olive oil, and lemon juice into a blender and puree.
2. Pour into a small saucepan and gently warm over a low heat. Set aside.
3. Pour the olive oil into a large pan and place this over medium heat.
4. Cook the onions in the olive oil until slightly transparent.

5. Pour in the chicken broth and orange juice.
6. Increase the heat and bring the mixture to a boil
7. Add the florets and cook them until crispy.
8. Remove the pan from the heat.
9. Puree the mixture in a blender.
10. Pour the puree back into the pan and keep warm until it is ready to serve.
11. When about to serve, use a ladle to pour the soup into serving bowls.
12. Pour some of the red pepper puree in dollops over the soup.
13. Using a knife, trace the dollops to get the pattern you want.
14. Serve while warm.

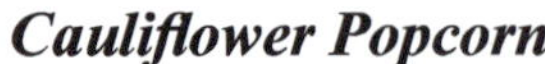

Cauliflower Popcorn

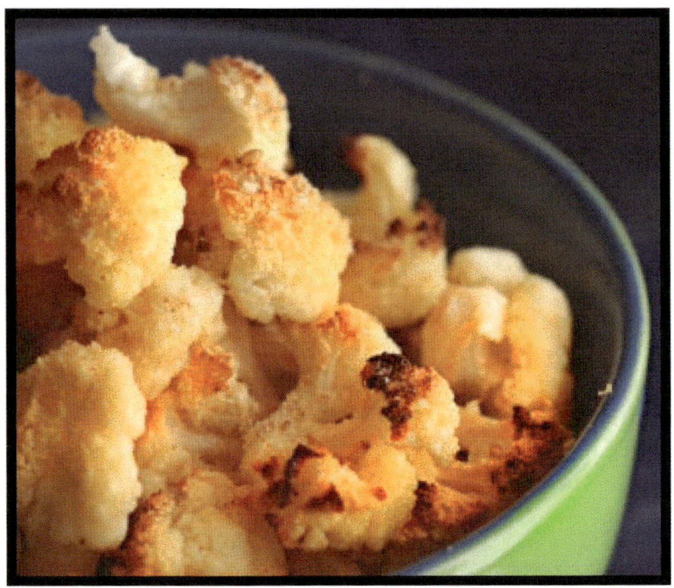

Ingredients:

1 head cauliflower
4 tbsp. olive oil
1 tsp. salt

Procedure:

1. Preheat the oven to 425°F
2. Shred the cauliflower head. Make sure to discard the core and thicker stems.
3. Cut the florets into bite-sized pieces
4. Mix the olive oil and salt in a large bowl.
5. Add the florets to the mixture and toss vigorously. Make sure to get an even coating on the florets.
6. Spread the coated florets on a baking sheet.
7. Roast the florets for about an hour. You should turn them 3 or 4 times for the entire duration.
8. Pull them out of the oven when they are a golden brown.

9. Pour in a serving bowl and enjoy immediately.

Charming Chicken Cacciatore

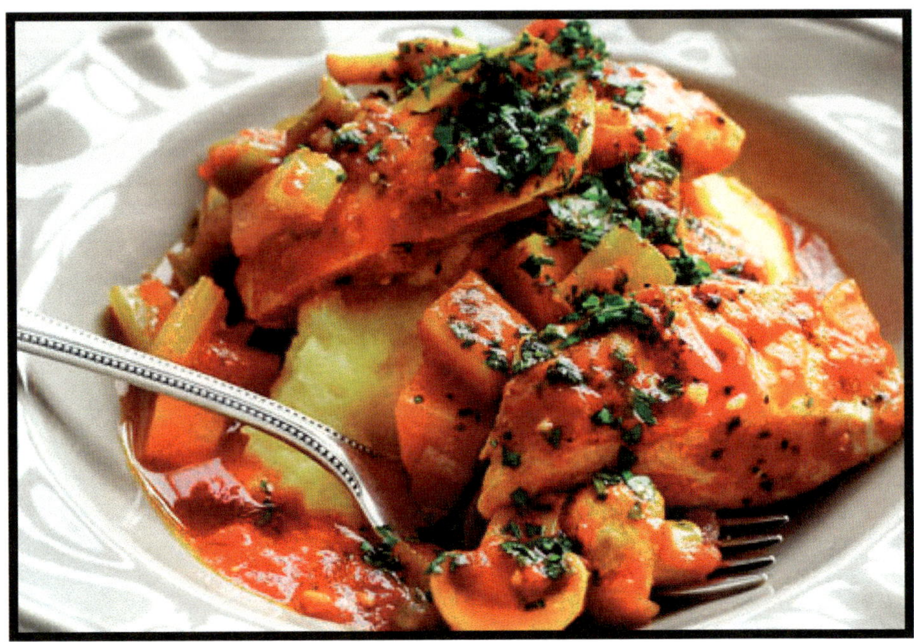

Ingredients:

- 1 ½ cup marinara sauce
- ½ cup onions, thinly sliced
- ¼ cup tomato paste
- ¼ cup red wine
- ½ tsp. rosemary
- ½ tsp. sea salt
- 8 chicken thighs, skinned
- 8 oz. mushrooms, quartered

Procedure:

1. In a large bowl, combine the marinara sauce, onions, tomato paste, wine, rosemary, and salt.
2. Pour this mixture into a slow cooker.
3. Add the chicken thighs and mushrooms.
4. Give a good toss to evenly coat each of the pieces.

5. Cook for 3 ½ hours on high, or 8 hours on low. You will know it's done when the chicken is tender.
6. Plate, garnish, and serve while warm.

Chicken and Vegetable Soup

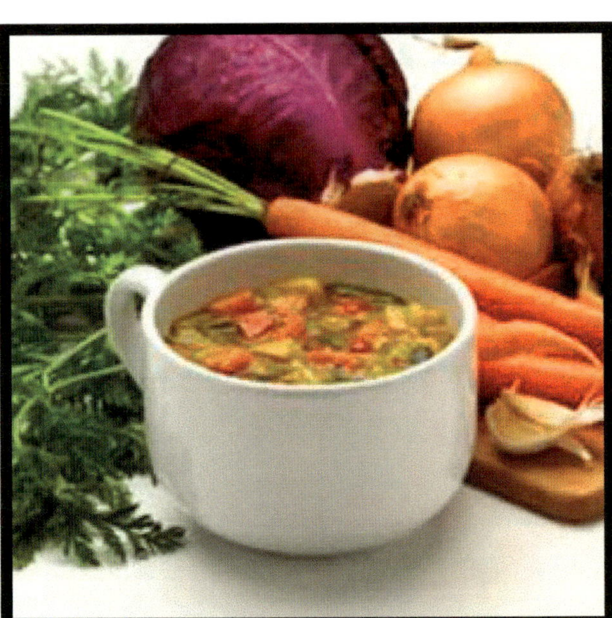

Ingredients:

12 oz. chicken breast
½ cup cabbage, chopped
1 large carrot, chopped
1 onion, chopped
2 celery stocks, diced
1 large can tomatoes, crushed
10 ¾ oz. can chicken broth
½ tsp. sea salt
¼ tsp. black pepper

Directions

1. Preheat the oven to 400°F.
2. Bake the chicken until thoroughly done.
3. Cut the cooked chicken into bite-sized chunks. Set aside.

4. Place all other ingredients into a fairly large pan.
5. Cook under over medium heat.
6. Let simmer for one hour, or until vegetables start to turn soft.
7. Add the chicken, and cook under reduced heat.
8. Serve while still warm.

Creamy Broccoli Soup

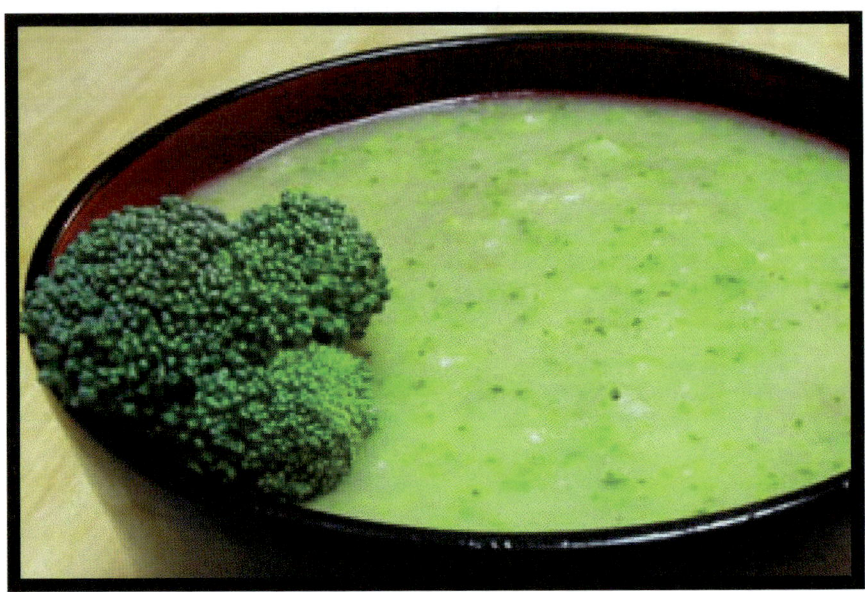

Ingredients:

2 tbsp. olive oil
2 cloves garlic, minced
1 yellow onion, chopped
½ red pepper, chopped
1 head broccoli, chopped
2 ½ cups chicken stock
Sea salt and black pepper to taste
Optional: lemon juice

Procedure:

1. Preheat a pan over medium heat.
2. Pour the olive oil on the pan.
3. Sauté the garlic, red pepper and onion.
4. Add the broccoli and cook for another 4 minutes before adding the stock.
5. Season with sea salt and black pepper to taste.

6. Bring the mixture to a boil.
7. Turn down the heat and let simmer for another 7 minutes.
8. Blend the mixture using a hand mixer.
9. Optionally, you may add some freshly squeezed lemon juice.
10. Serve while still hot.

Crispy Kale Chips

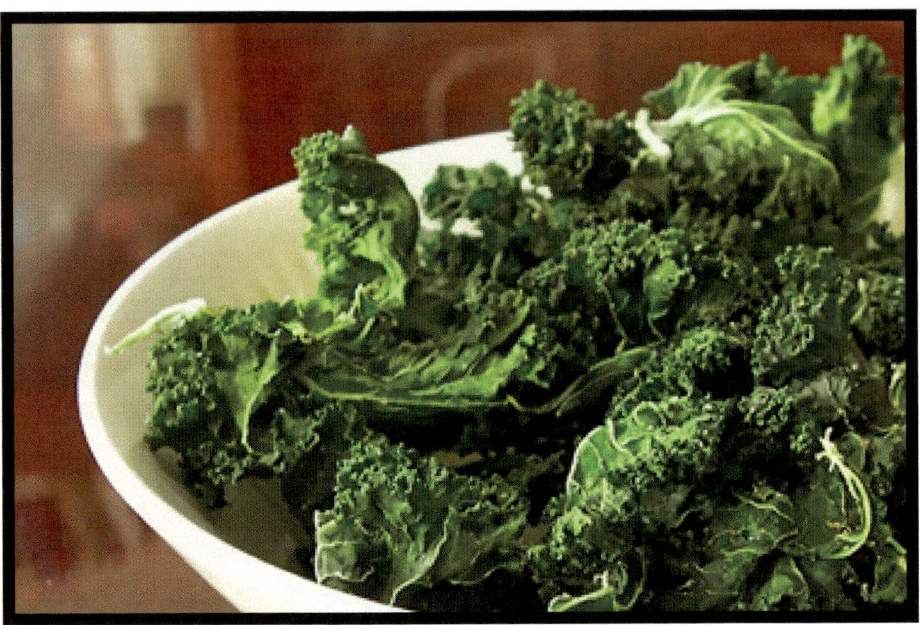

Ingredients:

2 cups kale leaves
2 tsp. olive oil
1 tsp. vinegar
1 tsp. soy sauce
Sea salt to taste

Procedure:

1. Preheat the oven to 350°F.
2. Wash the kale leaves and tear them into small pieces.
3. Place these pieces in a large bowl and set aside.
4. In a small bowl, mix the olive oil, vinegar, and soy sauce.
5. Pour the contents into the bowl of kale.
6. Toss vigorously to coat each leaf.
7. Spread the kale on a cookie sheet.
8. Bake for 10 minutes before stirring the contents of the sheet.

9. Bake for another 12 minutes or until kale turns crispy. It should crackle when touched and be dark green in color.
10. Remove from oven and place in a clean large bowl.
11. Season with sea salt to taste before serving.

Delectable Carrot Fries

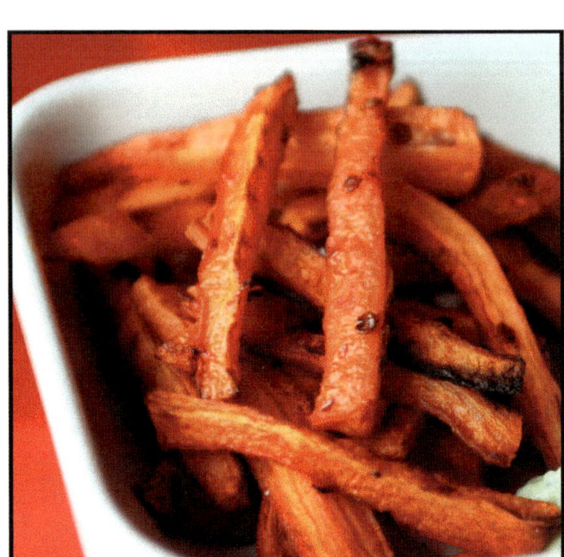

Ingredients:

4 large carrots
All-spice to taste
Optional: sea salt, ketchup, or mayonnaise

Procedure:

1. Peel the carrots.
2. Cut them into 2 inch pieces.
3. Season the pieces with all-spice
4. Cook the pieces until a little tender, but still crispy.
5. Let the pieces cool a bit before serving.
6. You may also opt to season the cooked pieces with sea salt to taste, or serve them with a dip like ketchup or mayonnaise.

Delicious Baked Salmon

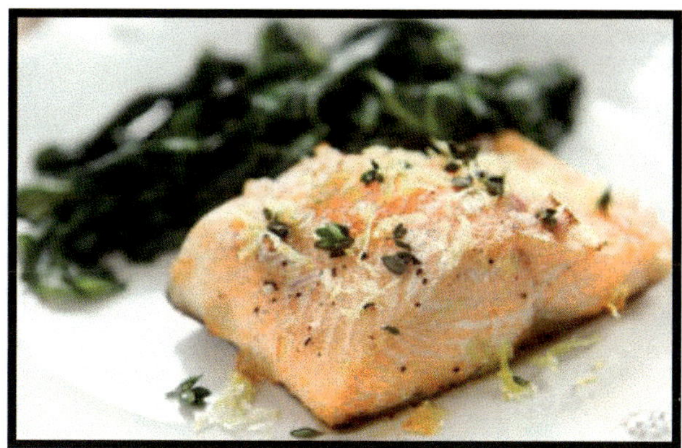

Ingredients:

2 cloves garlic
2 tbsp. olive oil
1 tsp. basil
1 tsp. sea salt
½ tsp. black pepper
1 tbsp. lemon juice
1 tbsp. parsley
2 fillets salmon

Procedure:

1. Mince the garlic and chop the parsley.
2. In a bowl, mix the garlic, sea salt, black pepper, basil, parsley olive oil, and lemon juice.
3. Put the salon in a Ziploc bag and pour in the contents of the bowl.
4. Refrigerate the bag for about an hour to marinate. Remember to turn the bag every now and then to evenly coat the fillets.
5. Preheat the oven to 375°F.
6. Remove the bag from the refrigerator.
7. Wrap the marinated fillets in aluminum foil.
8. Before sealing the foil, pour some of the marinade over the fillets.
9. Bake until the fillets flake easily with a fork.
10. Plate, garnish, and serve.

Egg and Turkey Scramble

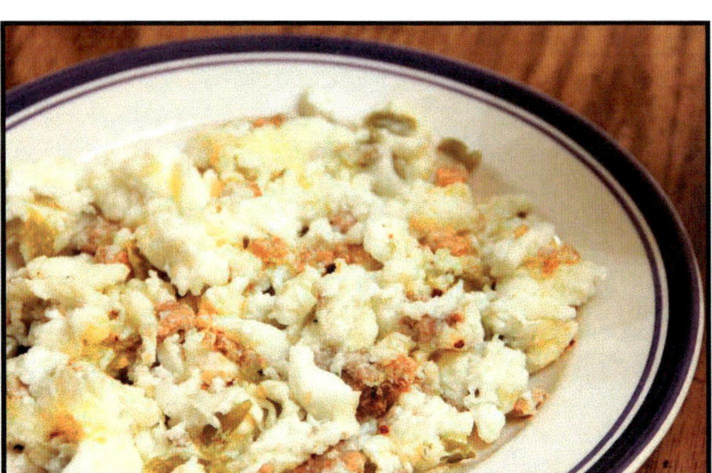

Ingredients:

8 egg whites
1 lb. lean turkey meat, ground
2 cups spinach, shredded
2 tomatoes
1 clove garlic, minced
Non-stick cooking spray
Sea salt and black pepper

Procedure:

1. Put the turkey meat in a skillet.
2. Cook over a medium heat until light brown. There may be excess juices from the pan, drain them before proceeding to the next step.
3. Get a large bowl and place the cooked turkey inside.
4. Pour boiling water over the bowl, and drain immediately after. This will reduce the further reduce the turkey's fat content.
5. Clean the skillet thoroughly, and wipe excess water off.
6. Scramble the egg whites in the skillet until thoroughly cooked.
7. Add the cooked egg whites to the turkey.
8. Clean the skillet thoroughly, and wipe excess water off.

9. Coat the skillet with the cooking spray.
10. Sauté the tomatoes, spinach, and garlic.
11. Add the sautéed vegetables to the turkey and eggs.
12. Evenly mix all the contents of the bowl.
13. Season with sea salt and black pepper.
14. Enjoy immediately.

Garlic and Spinach Soup

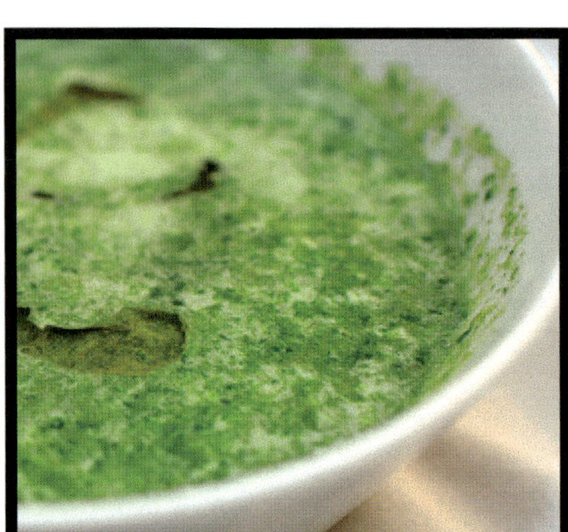

Ingredients:

2 heads garlic, peeled
2 tsp. virgin olive oil
5 cups vegetable broth
3 cups spinach leaves, chopped.

Procedure:

1. Preheat the oven to 425°F
2. Slice the heads in such a way that most of the cloves are exposed.
3. Place the sliced garlic in a small baking dish.
4. Drizzle 1 tsp. of olive oil over each head.
5. Cover the baking dish with aluminum foil.
6. Roast the garlic heads for 45 minutes.
7. Set aside and let cool.
8. Preheat a saucepan over medium heat.
9. Squeeze garlic pulp into a saucepan.
10. Add the broth and stir briskly.
11. Let simmer for 15 minutes.
12. Add the spinach leaves and simmer for 4 minutes, or until the leaves

wilt. Remember to stir vigorously.

13. Ladle over serving bowls.
14. Serve immediately.

Golden Onion Rings

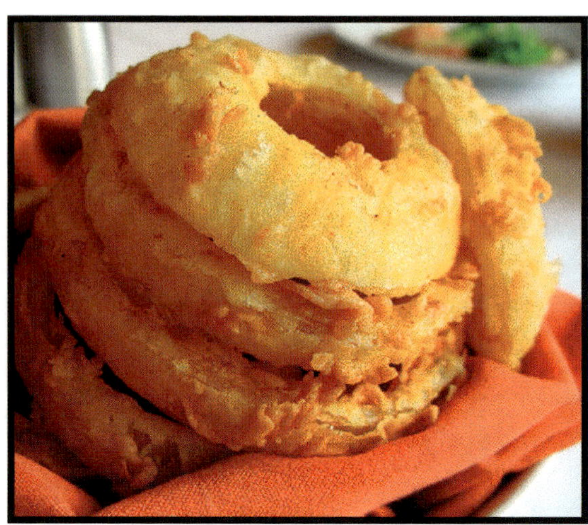

Ingredients:

6 slices sweet onion
2 egg whites
1 tbsp. hot sauce
2 tbsp. fat-free parmesan
1 pinch of garlic powder
Olive oil

Directions:

1. Spray a cookie sheet with some olive oil.
2. Preheat the oven to 400°F.
3. In a small bowl, beat the egg whites with the hot sauce. Make sure you do it lightly.
4. Dip the onions into the small bowl, making sure to evenly coat them with the mixture inside.
5. Place each coated ring on the prepared cookie sheet. Repeat the process until all 6 rings are coated.
6. Sprinkle the cheese onto each piece.
7. Spray more olive oil on the onion slices.
8. Bake the onion rings for 15 minutes. Remember to turn them once to get them to cook evenly.
9. Serve them with a mayonnaise dip.

Juicy Tuna Steaks

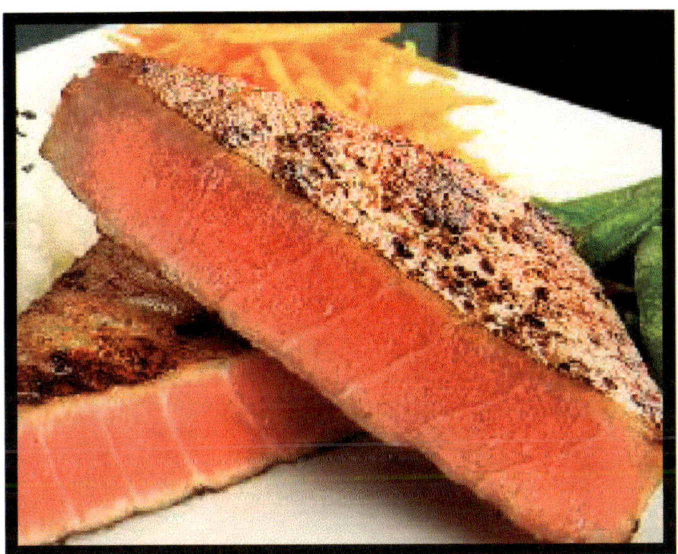

Ingredients:

1 fresh tuna steak
Steak seasoning
Non-stick cooking spray

Procedure:

1. Rub each steak with the steak seasoning and let sit for 5 minutes.
2. Coat a skillet with the cooking spray.
3. Preheat the skillet over a medium-high heat.
4. Place the steaks on the skillet.
5. Sear each side, but leave the middle slightly pink.
6. Serve with a side of steamed vegetables.
7. Enjoy!

Lemon Chicken

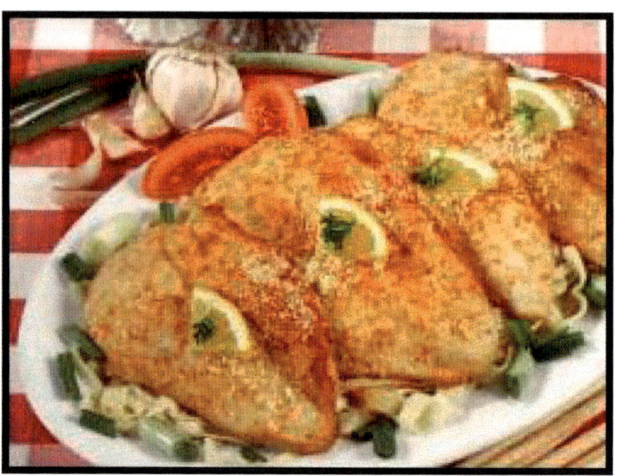

Ingredients:

- 1 ½ lb. chicken breast
- ½ cup lemon juice
- 2 tbsp. vinegar
- ½ cup lemon peel
- 3 tsp. fresh oregano
- 1 onion
- ¼ tsp. sea salt
- ½ tsp. paprika
- ¼ tsp. black pepper

Procedure:

1. Skin the chicken breasts.
2. Place the chicken breasts in a 9x13 baking pan.
3. Slice the lemon peel and onion. Crush the oregano.
4. In a small bowl, mix the lemon juice and peel, oregano, and onions.
5. Pour the contents of the small bowl over the chicken breasts.
6. Cover the baking pan and refrigerate overnight. Remember to turn the chicken breasts every now and then to get an even coating.
7. Preheat the oven to 325°F.
8. Remove the cover and sprinkle with the sea salt, paprika, and black

pepper.

9. Cover the baking pan again and bake for 30 minutes.
10. Best enjoyed when fresh out of the oven.

Lemon Turkey Cutlets

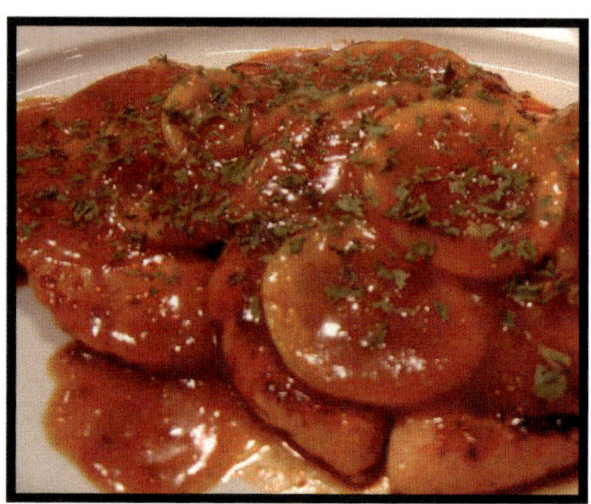

Ingredients:
1 lb. turkey cutlets
½ tsp. sea salt
1 tsp. black pepper
2 lemons
1 cup chicken broth
2 tsp. cornstarch
1 tbsp. olive oil
2 cloves garlic, crushed
2 tbsp. parsley, chopped

Procedure:

1. Use plastic wrap to cover the turkey cutlets. Tenderize them with a rolling pin until ¼ inch thick.
2. Remove the plastic wrap and season the cutlets with salt and pepper.
3. Grate peel one lemon to make ½ tsp. zest.
4. Halve one lemon. Grate peel one half to make ½ tsp. zest. Squeeze the other to make tbsp. juice.
5. Thinly slice the other lemon.
6. In a small bowl, thoroughly mix the chicken broth and cornstarch.

Set aside.
7. Pour the olive oil in a skillet and place it over high heat.
8. Sauté the turkey cutlets for 3 minutes on each side.
9. Plate the cutlets and set aside.
10. Add the lemon juice, zest, slices, and garlic to the skillet.
11. Stir briskly and cook for 30 seconds.
12. Pour the contents of the small bowl into the skillet.
13. Reduce the heat to medium and boil for 1 minute.
14. Pour the resulting mixture over the plated turkey cutlets.
15. Serve while warm.

Oriental Chicken Salad

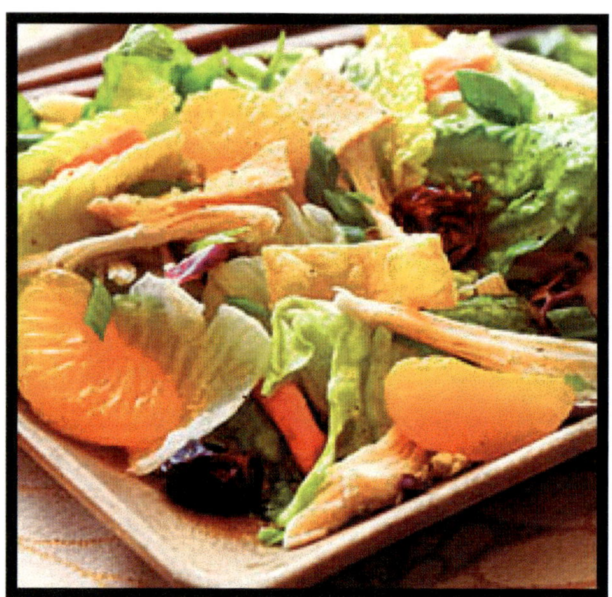

Ingredients:

2 cups chicken, skinned, cooked, and chopped
4 cups cabbage
1 cup mushrooms
1 cup carrots
2 tbsp. cilantro
1 cucumber
3 green onions
1 tangerine, peeled and sectioned
½ cup oriental salad dressing
Sea salt and black pepper to taste

Procedure:

1. Shred the cabbage. Slice the mushrooms. Grate the carrots. Chop the cilantro. Thinly slice the cucumber, and green onions.
2. Combine all the ingredients, except the green onions and tangerine, in a large bowl. Add the salad dressing last and mix evenly.

3. Top the salad with the green onions and tangerine.
4. Season with sea salt and pepper to taste. Some people prefer to not add salt at all.
5. Enjoy fresh!

Quick and Easy Chicken Creole

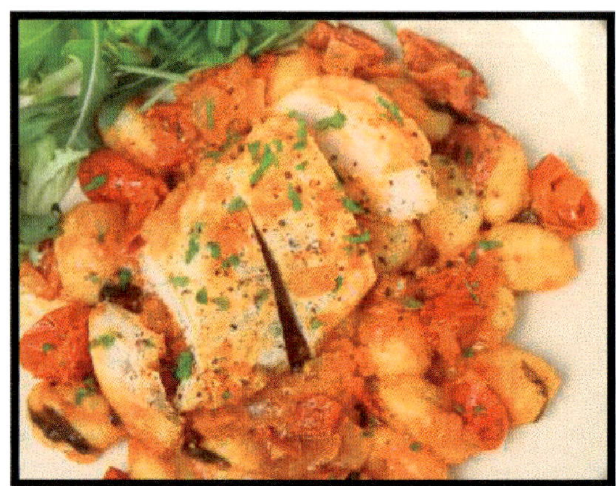

Ingredients:

- 4 Boneless chicken breasts
- 1 14oz. can tomatoes
- 1 ½ cups green peppers
- ½ cup celery
- 1 tbsp. fresh parsley
- 2 cloves garlic
- 1 tbsp. fresh basil
- ¼ cup onion
- ¼ tsp. red pepper
- ¼ tsp. sea salt
- Non-stick cooking spray

Procedure:

1. Coat a skillet with the cooking spray.
2. Preheat the skillet with high heat.
3. Skin the chicken breast, and cut them into 1 inch strips.
4. Cut up the canned tomatoes.
5. Chop the green peppers, celery, and onion. Mince the garlic cloves. Crush the red peppers.
6. In the skillet, cook the chicken breasts for 5 minutes or until they turn a golden brown. Make sure to stir continuously. When done, reduce the heat.

7. Add the cut up tomatoes including their juice, celery, onion, minced garlic, crushed red pepper, basil, sea salt, parsley, and green peppers.
8. Bring the mixture to a boil. Reduce the heat, and let it simmer while covered. Leave it for around 10 minutes.
9. Serve while hot.

Roasted Carrot and Garlic Soup

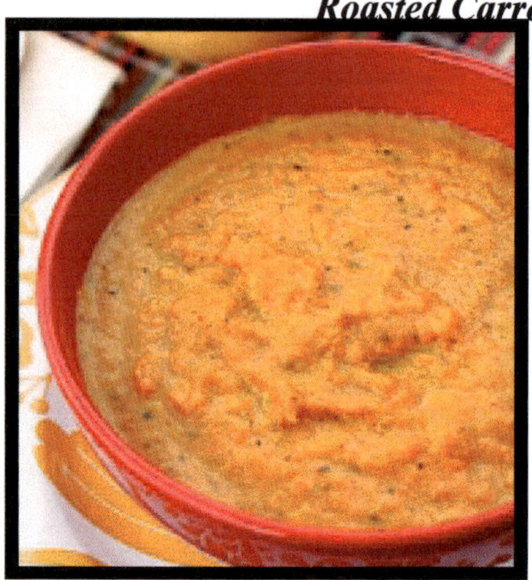

Ingredients:

2 lbs. carrots, peeled
1 yellow onion, sliced thinly
1 head garlic
1 tbsp. olive oil
3 tbsp. canola pol
1 tbsp. butter, melted
2 cups chicken stock
2 tsp. cumin powder
Sea salt and black pepper to taste

Procedure:

1. Preheat the oven to 300°F
2. Cut off the top third of the garlic head.
3. Drizzle with the olive oil and wrap in aluminum foil. Place in a small baking pan.
4. In a large baking pan, arrange the carrots in a single layer.
5. Pour canola oil over them, and stir so each piece is evenly coated.
6. Roast the carrots and garlic in the oven for 1 hour.
7. Stir the carrots every 20 minutes to prevent sticking.
8. In a large skillet, heat the butter over a medium-low heat.
9. Sauté the onion slices for 15 minutes.

10. Turn off the heat and wait for the carrots to finish roasting.
11. Remove the garlic from the oven, unwrap, and set aside to cool.
12. Turn up the ovens heat to 350°F.
13. Continue roasting the carrots for 15 minutes.
14. Add the carrots to the onions along with 2 cups of stock.
15. Turn the heat to medium and let simmer for 15 minutes. When done, place them in a blender.
16. Squeeze out bulbs of garlic and place them in the blender along with the carrots and onions. Blend until the mixture is smooth.
17. Pour the soup back into the skillet and let simmer.
18. Season with cumin, sea salt, and black pepper.
19. Ladle into serving bowls and enjoy while hot.

Roasted Garlic and Parmesan Soup

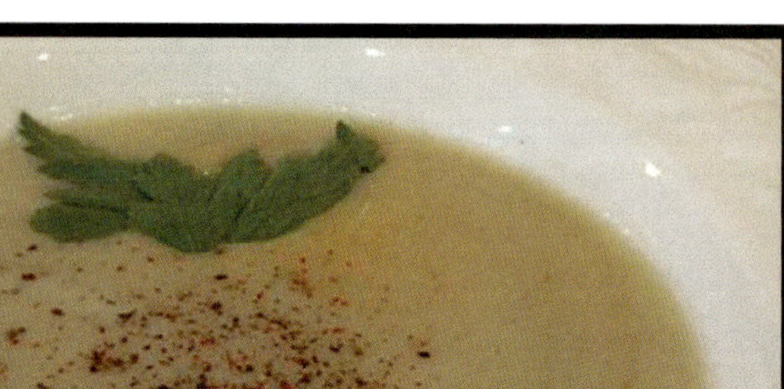

Ingredients:

26 cloves garlic, roasted
2 tbsp. olive oil
2 tbsp. butter, melted
2 ¼ cups onions, sliced
1 ½ tsp. thyme, chopped
18 cloves garlic, peeled
3 ½ cups chicken stock
½ cup whipping cream
½ cup parmesan cheese, grated
1 small lemon, quartered
Sea salt and black pepper to taste

Procedure:

1. In a large saucepan, cook the melted butter, onions, and thyme over a medium-high heat for 6 minutes.
2. Add all the garlic, roasted and peeled. Cook for another 3 minutes.
3. Pour in the chicken stock. Cover and let simmer for 20 minutes, or

until the garlic turns tender.

4. Pour the contents of the saucepan into a large bowl.
5. Use a blender to puree the soup.
6. Pour the pureed soup back into the saucepan.
7. Add the cream and let simmer.
8. Season with sea salt and black pepper.
9. Prepare four small serving bowls and divide the cheese among them.
10. Ladle the soup into the bowls.
11. Squeeze each quarter of lemon into a bowl before serving.

Special Thai Chicken

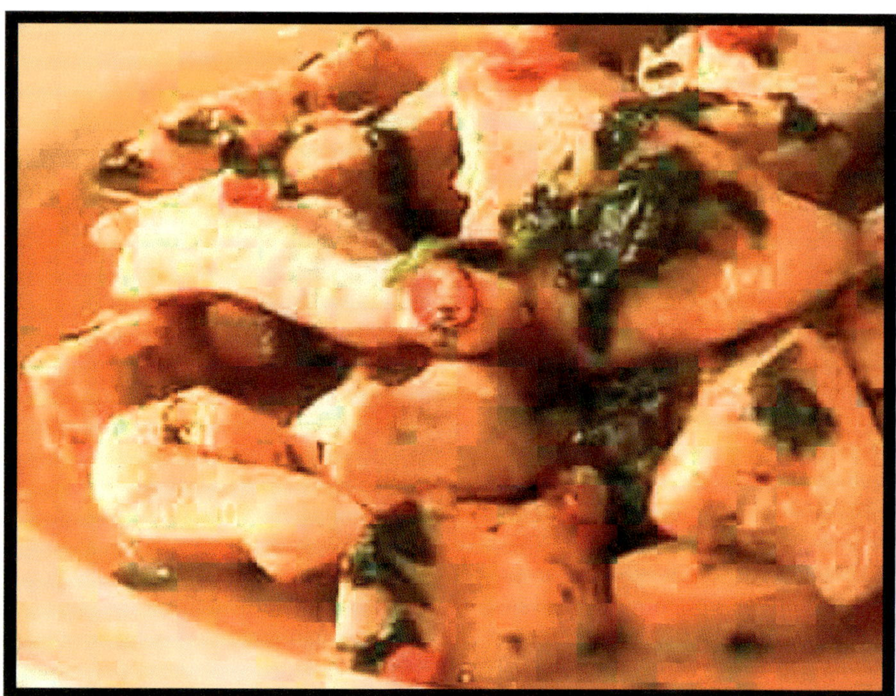

Ingredients:

2 boneless chicken breasts, skinned
½ cup salsa
1 tbsp. lime juice
½ tbsp. soy sauce
½ tsp. ginger
1 pinch black pepper
1 cilantro, chopped
1 scallion, chopped
Non-stick cooking spray

Procedure:

1. Set aside the chicken and combine all the other ingredients in a

medium bowl.

2. Pour the contents of the bowl over the chicken.
3. Coat a pan with the cooking spray.
4. Place the coated chicken into this pan.
5. Cook over low heat until the chicken breast is no longer pink.

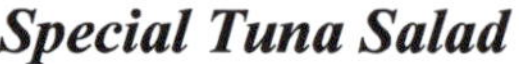

Special Tuna Salad

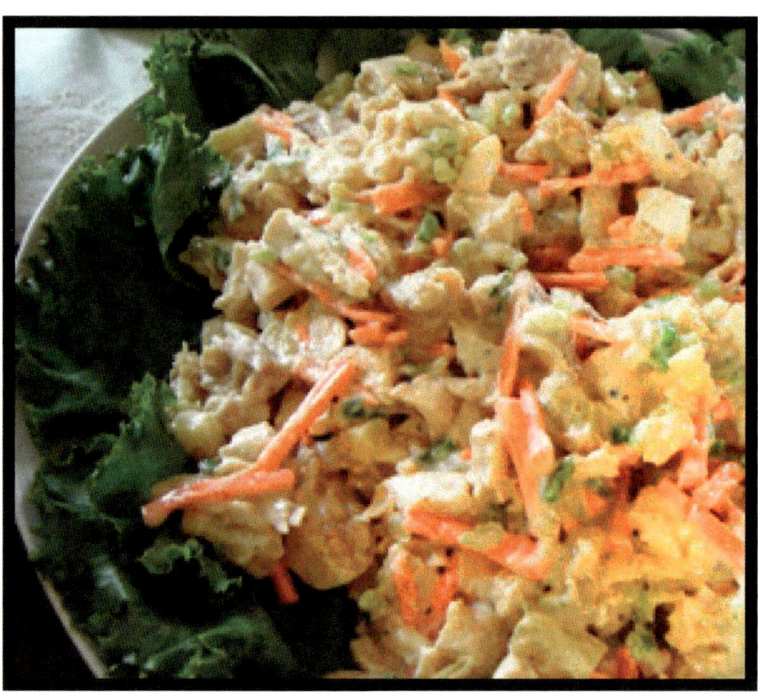

Ingredients:

- 1 can of tuna
- 1 cup red onions
- ¼ cup red pepper
- 2 egg whites, hard boiled
- 1 carrot, large
- 3 tbsp. mayonnaise
- Sea salt and black pepper

Procedure:

1. Cut up the dry ingredients. Alternatively, you may also use a food processor.
2. Mix the processed ingredients and mayonnaise in a large bowl.

3. Give the salad a good toss.
4. Season with sea salt and black pepper to taste.
5. Enjoy!

Spicy Turkey Burgers

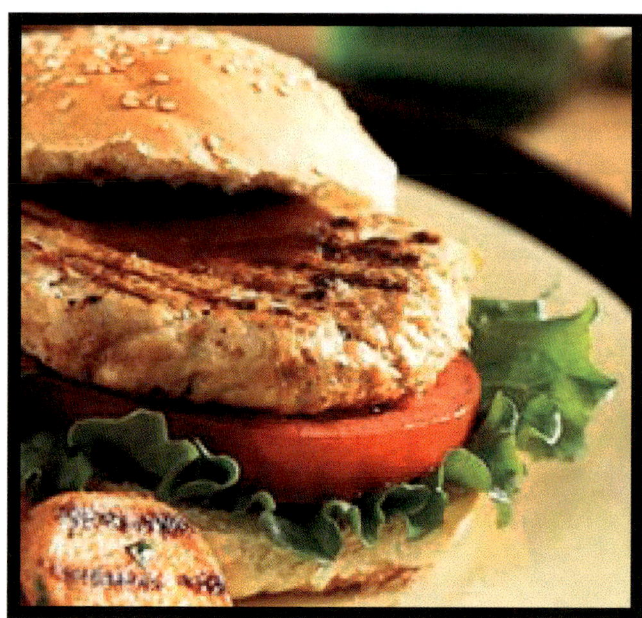

Ingredients:

- 1 ¼ lbs. lean turkey, ground
- 1 tsp. sea salt
- 1 tsp. cumin powder
- 1 tsp. garlic powder
- ½ tsp. black pepper
- 1 tbsp. chipotle chile in adobo
- ¼ cup red onion, chopped
- ½ cup cilantro leaves, chopped

Procedure:

1. In a large bowl, combine all the ingredients.
2. Scoop out the mixture and divide into 4 burger patties.
3. Grill the patties until thoroughly cooked.
4. Make a burger out of each patty.
5. Optionally, you may tomatoes or lettuce.
6. Indulge!

Spicy Turkey Chili

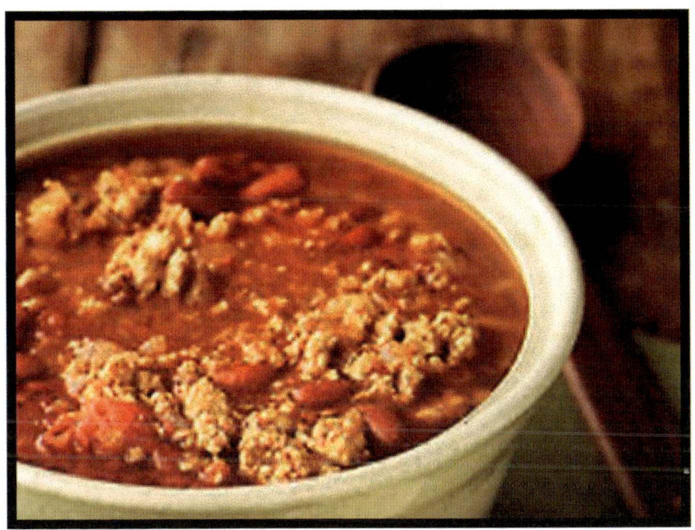

Ingredients:

1 lb. lean turkey, ground
1 white onion, diced
3 cloves garlic, minced
1 can tomatoes, crushed
1 tbsp. cumin
1 tbsp. chili powder
1 tbsp. white pepper, ground

Procedure:

1. In a large pan over medium heat, cook the turkey and onions until light brown. Add the garlic as you cook.
2. Season the mixture with the cumin, chili powder, and white pepper.
3. Add the can of tomatoes.
4. Continue cooking over a med-low heat for 20 minutes. This should let the flavors develop more deeply.
5. Pour into a serving bowl.
6. Enjoy!

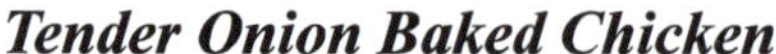

Tender Onion Baked Chicken

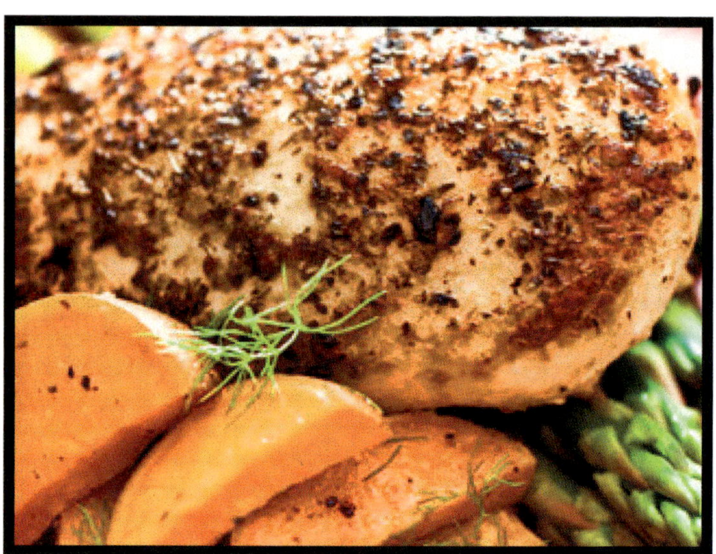

Ingredients:

- 2 chicken breasts
- 1 tbsp. butter
- ½ cup water
- 1 pack onion soup mix
- Sea salt and black pepper

Procedure:

1. Preheat the oven to 350°F
2. Melt the butter.
3. Set the chicken breasts in a 9x13 baking pan.
4. Pour the melted butter over the chicken breasts.
5. Season with sea salt and black pepper to taste.
6. Sprinkle with the onion soup mix.
7. Bake the chicken breasts until no longer pink. You'll know they are done when their juices run clear. This will take around 35 minutes.
8. Garnish and serve.

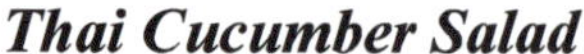

Thai Cucumber Salad

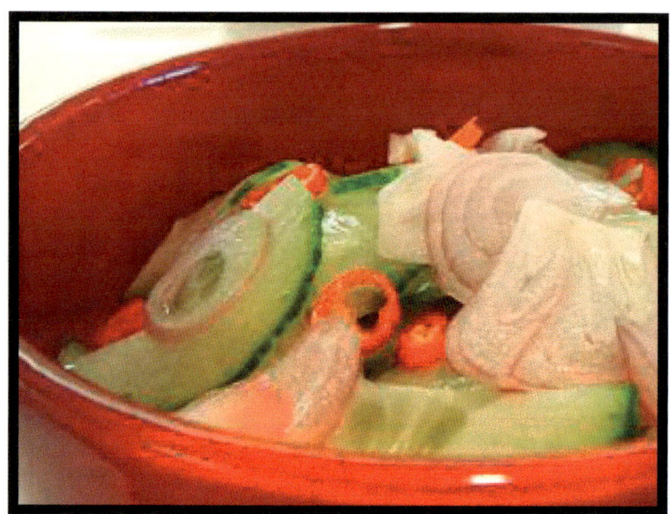

Ingredients:

- 1 cucumber
- ½ red onion
- 1 jalapeno pepper
- 1 tbsp. red pepper flakes
- 2 tbsp. cilantro
- 3 tbsp. vinegar
- 3 tbsp. lime juice
- 2 tbsp. water
- 2 packs artificial sweetener
- ½ tsp. sea salt

Procedure:

1. Slice and seed the cucumber. Slice the onion into thin pieces. Chop the jalapeno pepper and the cilantro.
2. Mix the water, lime juice, vinegar, sea salt, artificial sweetener, and red pepper flakes in a small bowl.
3. In a larger serving bowl arrange the layers of the salad in the following order: cucumber, jalapeno pepper, cilantro and onion.

4. Pour the contents of the small bowl into the serving bowl.
5. Place the serving bowl in the fridge for 30 minutes.
6. When cool, toss the salad.
7. Enjoy!

Traditional Fried Rice

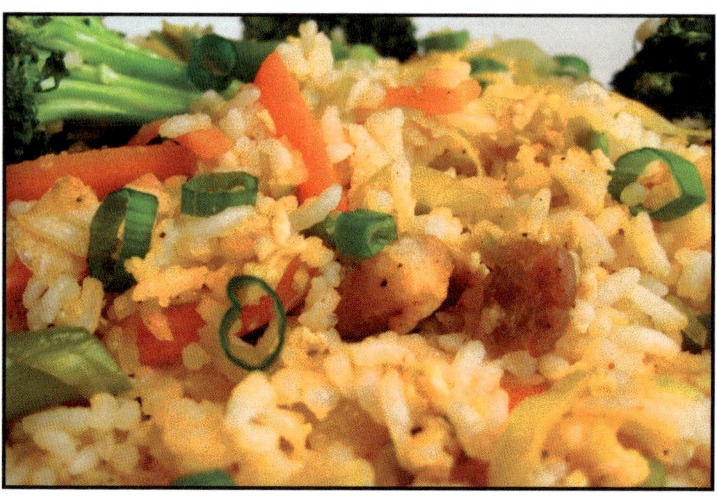

Ingredients:

1 lb. boneless chicken breast, skinned, and chopped
½ head cauliflower
3 green onions, chopped
¼ tsp. ginger, grated
1 clove garlic, minced
1 cup cooked rice
1 egg
2 tsp. soy sauce
Non-stick cooking pray
Optional: carrots, bean sprouts, chopped celery

Procedure:

1. Spray a skillet with the cooking spray.
2. Sauté the chicken breast until done. Set aside on a plate.
3. Shred the cauliflower head and sauté in the same skillet.
4. Add the garlic, onion, ginger, and rice. If you also want to use some of the optional ingredients, now is the time to add them.
5. Cook for 5 minutes.
6. Push everything to the sides of the skillet.

7. Crack the egg and pour the contents right into the center of the skillet.
8. Scramble it, and mix it in with the other ingredients as it cooks.
9. Add the chicken breast and the soy sauce.
10. Place the contents of the skillet on a plate and top with green onions.
11. Serve while still hot.

Zesty Garlic Chicken

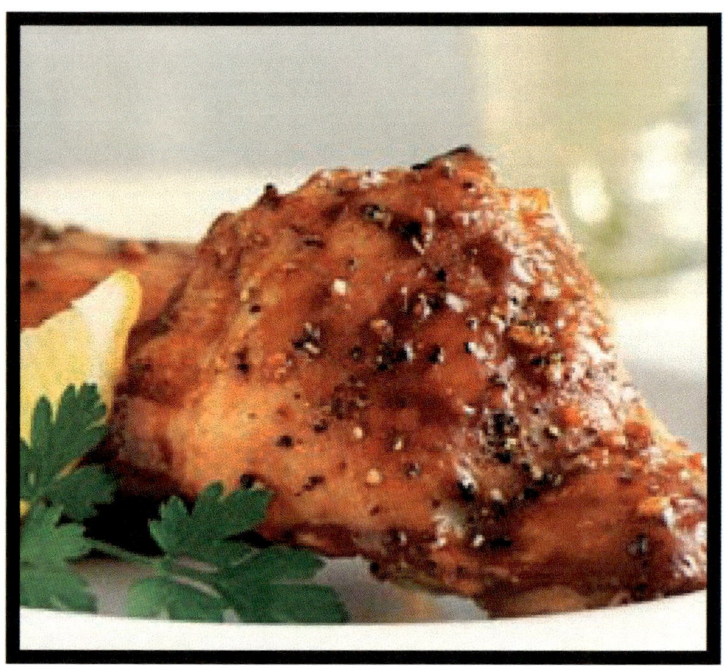

Ingredients:

4 boneless chicken breasts, skinned
¼ tsp. salt
¼ tsp. pepper
40 cloves garlic, halved
1 tbsp. olive oil
1 cup chicken broth
1 tbsp. lemon juice
1 tsp. basil
½ tsp. oregano
4 tsp. flour
2 tbsp. white wine

Procedure:

1. Season the chicken breasts on each side with the salt and pepper.

2. In a large pan, cook the chicken breasts in the olive oil until light brown.
3. Pour in the lemon juice, chicken broth, oregano, and basil.
4. Increase the heat and bring the soup to a boil.
5. Reduce the heat and cover the pan. Let the contents simmer for 9 minutes.
6. Remove the chicken and garlic from the pan.
7. Pour the wine and flour into the pan. Stir briskly.
8. Increase the heat and bring to a boil.
9. Cook the contents of the pan until they thicken.
10. Plate the chicken and garlic, and pour the resulting sauce over them.
11. Enjoy!

Heres to good health!

Recipes used from this book and prepared are done so "at your own risk." Robert Johnson is not responsible for any damage, medically or otherwise, resulting in the preparation of food using the instructions or recipes provided in this book. Readers must take care to check the instructions provided and determine their value and any possible medical condition that may arise from the consumption of the ingredients listed in this book

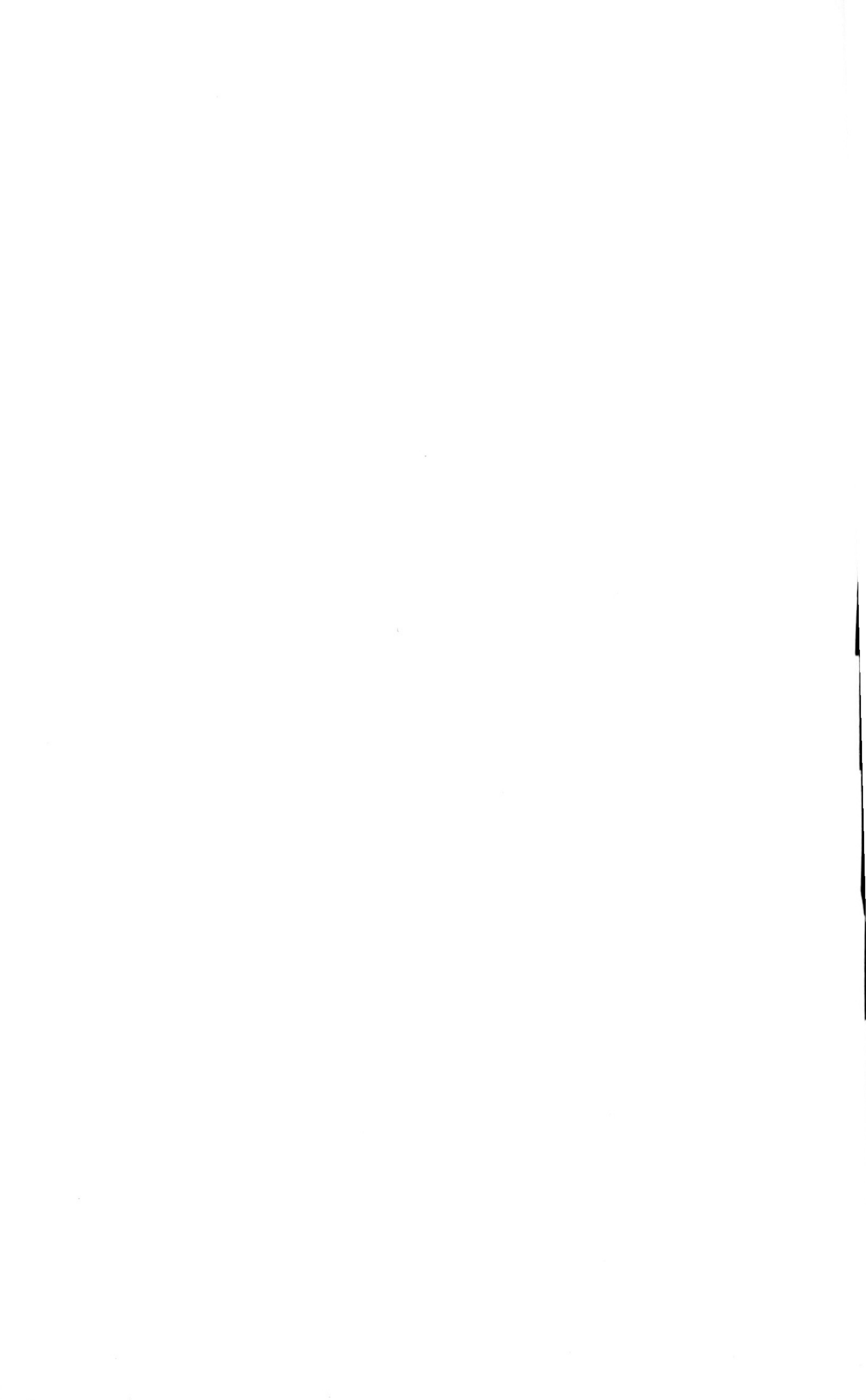

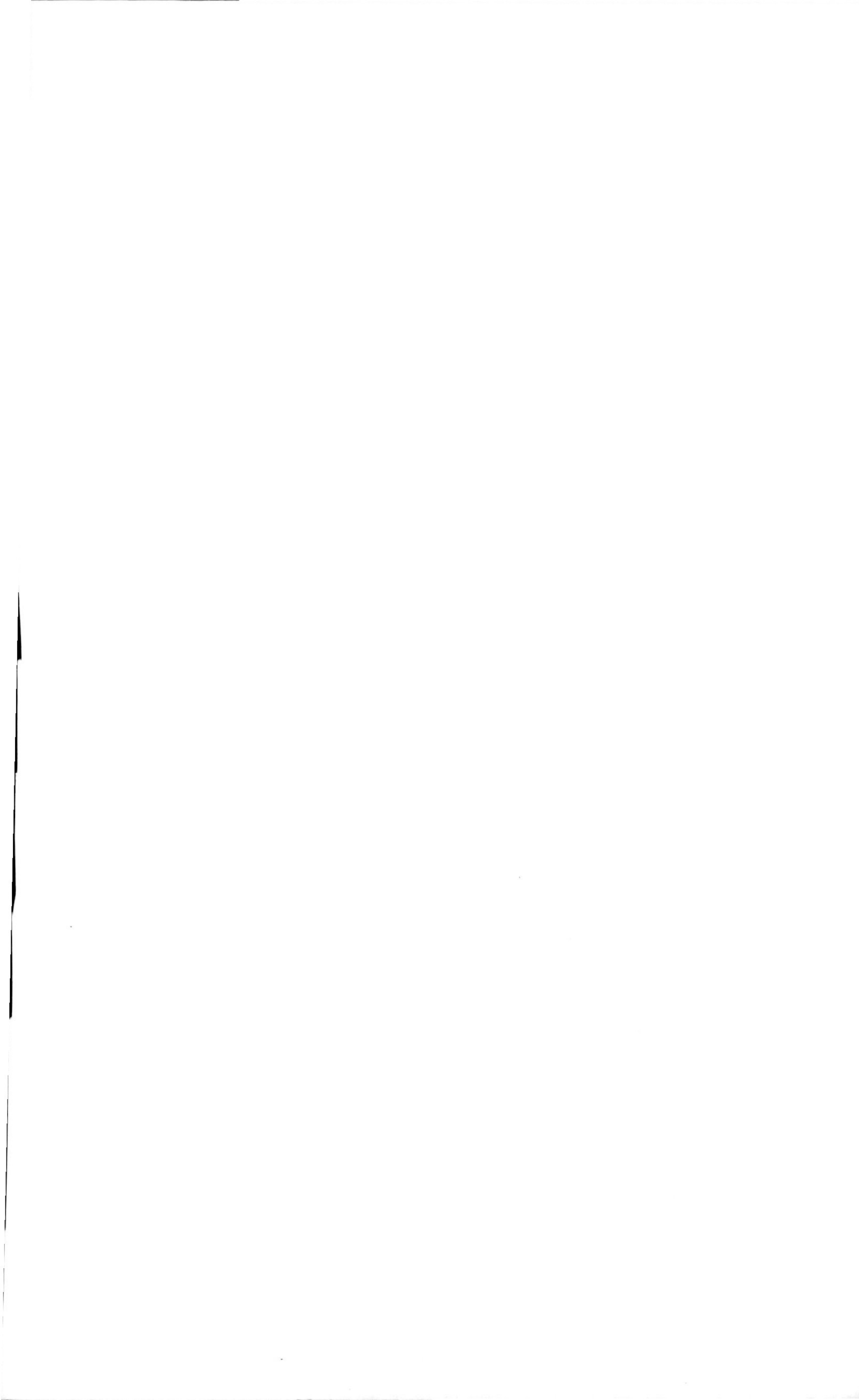

Made in the USA
Lexington, KY
09 January 2014